MORNING EXERCISES
FOR OLDER MEN OVER 50

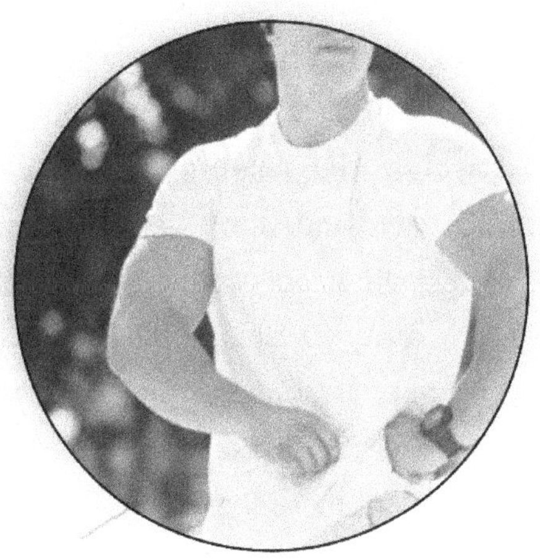

STRENGTHEN YOUR BODY AND IMPROVE YOUR BALANCE

Harry Lance

Abstract

A daily morning workout for older men is essential for maintaining physical and mental well-being. This tailored routine combines cardiovascular exercises, strength training, and flexibility exercises to cater to the unique needs of aging bodies.

Cardiovascular exercises like brisk walking or cycling improve heart health and overall stamina. Strength training, including bodyweight exercises and light weights, helps maintain muscle mass and bone density, combating age-related muscle loss and osteoporosis.

Incorporating flexibility exercises like yoga or stretching routines enhances joint mobility and reduces the risk of injury. Consistency is key, ensuring gradual progress and improved vitality, enabling older men to enjoy an active and fulfilling lifestyle as they age gracefully.

STRENGTHEN YOUR BODY AND IMPROVE YOUR BALANCE

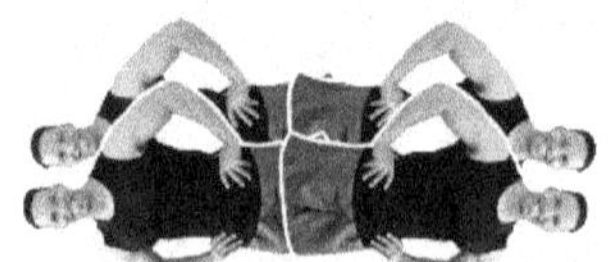

DON'T LET TIME DICTATE YOUR FITNESS, LET FITNESS DEFY TIME

TABLE OF CONTENT

Here are 15 morning workout exercises

FREE WORKOUT JOURNAL INCLUDED

INTRODUCTION

In a world that often seems obsessed with youth, there is a hidden treasure trove of wisdom and power that comes with experience. I'm Charles, a sixty-year-old man on a quest to share a three-month-old experience of transformation, vigor, and joy. I'm glad you're here. Thank you for reading "Ageless Vitality: A Blueprint for Lifelong Fitness."

They say that age is just a number, and I couldn't agree more. Our bodies and minds change significantly as we age, but this does not mean that we have to accept a sedentary, inactive existence. It's never too late to take charge of your health and wellbeing, in fact, in my opinion.

I chose to change my life three months ago. I started a daily exercise program designed especially for mature men like myself, and the results have been nothing short of amazing. I now have a new outlook on life, one that is characterized by an abundance of energy, a rekindled sense of purpose, and a level of enjoyment I haven't felt in a long time.

I'll walk you through this life-changing process in "Ageless Vitality," sharing the exercises, methods, and attitude adjustments that have not only helped me get fit but also rediscover my joy for living. This book is about more than just exercising; it's also about realizing your full potential, accepting age-related wisdom, and living a healthy, happy life. List 15 daily morning workout for older men for a successful workout

STRENGTHEN YOUR BODY AND IMPROVE YOUR BALANCE

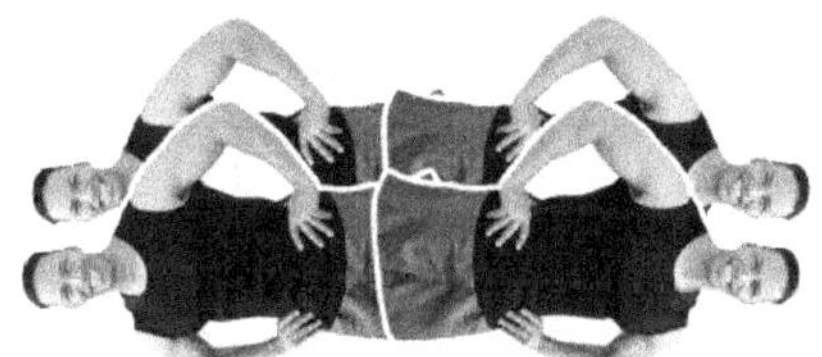

DON'T LET TIME DICTATE YOUR FITNESS, LET FITNESS DEFY TIME

Here are 15 morning workout exercises that can be beneficial for older men. Remember to consult a healthcare professional before starting a new workout routine, especially if you have any medical conditions.

1.WARM-UP

Warming up before a workout is crucial for individuals of all ages, but it becomes especially important as we get older. As we age, our muscles, joints, and cardiovascular system require more attention and care to ensure a safe and effective exercise routine. For older men, a proper warm-up is essential to prevent injuries, enhance flexibility, and optimize the benefits of a workout.

The warm-up phase is the initial step in any exercise routine, and it sets the stage for what follows. Older men should prioritize activities that gradually prepare the body for more intense exercises. A suitable warm-up generally consists of light aerobic exercises that increase heart rate, improve circulation, and engage major muscle groups.

To start a warm-up for older men, consider the following steps:

1. Assessment: Before beginning any exercise, it's essential to assess your current physical condition. Consult with a healthcare professional or fitness expert to identify any specific concerns or limitations. This assessment will help you tailor your warm-up routine to your individual needs.

2. Choose the Right Location: Find a safe and comfortable place to perform your warm-up. You can do it indoors or outdoors, as long as the environment is suitable for the chosen activities.

3. Appropriate Attire: Wear comfortable clothing and supportive footwear. Proper attire ensures you can move freely and reduces the risk of injury.

4. Light Aerobic Exercises: Start with light aerobic exercises that gradually increase your heart rate. These can include marching in place or gentle jumping jacks. Marching in place involves lifting your knees alternately as you walk in one spot, while gentle jumping jacks involve stepping out to the sides with minimal impact.

5. Duration: Aim for 5-10 minutes of light aerobic exercise. This duration allows your body to adapt to increased blood flow and prepares it for more intense movements.

6. Controlled breathing is the key throughout the warm-up. Breathe in slowly through your mouth after taking a big breath through your nose. This promotes relaxation and oxygenates your muscles.

7. Joint Mobility: As we age, joint mobility can become a concern. Incorporate gentle joint mobility exercises into your warm-up. Examples include ankle circles, wrist rotations, and shoulder shrugs. These movements improve flexibility and reduce the risk of strains.

8. Dynamic Stretches: Dynamic stretches involve controlled, active movements that mimic the upcoming workout's motions. For older men, dynamic stretches like leg swings, arm circles, and hip rotations are excellent choices. These stretches help prepare the muscles and reduce the risk of injury.

9. Gradual Progression: The warm-up should progressively increase in intensity but never push you to your limits. Listen to your body, and if you experience pain or discomfort, adjust the intensity or technique.

10. Hydration: Stay hydrated during your warm-up and throughout your workout. Proper hydration supports overall exercise performance and reduces the risk of cramps.

11. Mental Focus: Use this time to mentally prepare for your workout. Set specific goals for your exercise session, and visualize yourself achieving them.

12. Cool Down: After completing your warm-up, transition into your main workout gradually. Start with exercises of moderate intensity, gradually building up to more strenuous activities. After your workout, remember to cool down with gentle stretches to promote recovery and flexibility.

In conclusion, a well-planned warm-up is essential for older men embarking on a workout. It prepares the body physically and mentally, reduces the risk of injuries, and enhances the overall effectiveness of the exercise routine. By incorporating light aerobic exercises, joint mobility work, dynamic stretches, and proper hydration, older men can enjoy safer and more enjoyable workouts that support their health and fitness goals. Remember that individual needs and abilities may vary, so it's essential to tailor your warm-up routine to your specific circumstances. Always consult with a healthcare professional or fitness expert for personalized guidance and recommendations.

2. NECK TILTS

To begin Neck Tilts, a simple yet effective exercise suitable for older men, follow these steps carefully. Neck tilts are great for improving neck mobility and reducing stiffness. Here's a step-by-step guide:

1. Preparation: Find a quiet and comfortable place to stand or sit with proper posture. Keep your back straight and shoulders relaxed. If you're seated, sit on a stable chair with your feet flat on the ground.

2. Neutral Position: Start in a neutral position with your head in a straight and upright posture, looking straight ahead. This is your starting point.

3. Side Tilt: Bring your ear to your shoulder and gently incline your head to the right. Avoid raising your shoulder so that it touches your ear.
- Hold the tilt for 10-15 seconds while feeling a gentle stretch along the left side of your neck.
- Return your head to the neutral position.
- Repeat the same tilt to the left side, holding for the same duration.

4. Forward and Backward Tilt:

- Slowly tilt your head forward, aiming to bring your chin towards your chest. Don't force it; go only as far as is comfortable.
- Hold for 10-15 seconds, feeling a stretch along the back of your neck.
- Return your head to the neutral position.
- Now, tilt your head backward, gently looking up towards the ceiling.
- Hold for 10-15 seconds while feeling the stretch along the front of your neck.

5. Repetition: Perform each of these tilts (side, forward, and backward) 2-3 times, gradually increasing the duration of the stretch as your neck muscles loosen

6. Breathing: Throughout the workout, keep your breath even and deep. Use your nose to take in air, and your mouth to let it out.

7. Safety: Always perform neck tilts slowly and with control. Avoid any sudden or jerky movements to prevent injury.

8.Frequency: Incorporate neck tilts into your daily routine or workout regimen. It's an excellent exercise for maintaining neck flexibility and reducing tension.

9. Consultation: If you have any existing neck or spinal issues, consult with a healthcare professional or physical therapist before starting this or any exercise routine.

By following these steps, you can safely and effectively perform neck tilts as a part of your workout regimen for older men, promoting neck flexibility and overall well-being.

STRENGTHEN YOUR BODY AND IMPROVE YOUR BALANCE

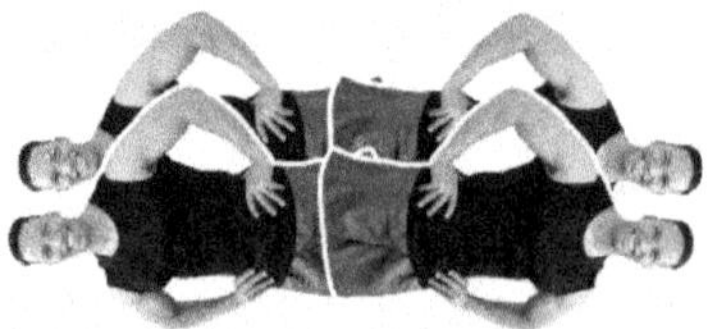

DON'T LET TIME DICTATE YOUR FITNESS, LET FITNESS DEFY TIME

3. SHOULDER ROLLS

To begin Shoulder Rolls, a simple yet effective exercise, follow these steps. This exercise is particularly beneficial for older men as it helps improve shoulder mobility and reduces stiffness.

1. Warm-Up: Before any exercise, it's crucial to warm up your body. Perform some light cardio exercises like brisk walking or gentle arm swings for about 5-10 minutes. This gets your blood flowing and prepares your muscles for movement.

2. Proper Posture: Stand up straight with your feet shoulder-width apart. Maintain good posture by keeping your spine aligned, and engage your core muscles slightly.

3. Relax Your Arms: Let your arms hang naturally at your sides. Keep your hands and fingers relaxed; there's no need to clench your fists.

4. Initiate the Movement: Start the shoulder roll by gently lifting your shoulders towards your ears. Imagine drawing a circle with your shoulders. This circular motion is what defines the exercise.

5. Rolling Motion: Continue rolling your shoulders in a forward direction, moving them forward, down, back, and up. Imagine that you're trying to touch your shoulders to your ears, then push them back and down, completing the circular motion.

6. Repetition: Perform this motion for about 10-15 seconds in a forward direction. You should feel a gentle stretch and loosening of the shoulder muscles.

7. Reverse Direction: After forward rolls, switch to rolling your shoulders in the reverse direction.
Lift your shoulders up, then move them back, down, and forward. Again, aim for 10-15 seconds.

8. Repeat as Needed: Depending on your comfort level and the tightness of your shoulder muscles, you can repeat this exercise for 1-3 sets. Remember to maintain a slow and controlled movement; don't rush.

9. Cool Down: After completing your sets, do some gentle neck stretches and deep breaths to relax your shoulders and bring your heart rate back to normal.
10.Frequency: You can perform shoulder rolls as part of your daily routine or before other workouts. Regular practice can lead to improved shoulder mobility and reduced muscle

tension, making it an excellent exercise for older men looking to stay active and flexible.

Remember to listen to your body. If you experience pain or discomfort, stop the exercise and consult a fitness professional or healthcare provider for guidance. Shoulder rolls should be a comfortable and gentle movement to promote shoulder health and mobility.

STRENGTHEN YOUR BODY AND IMPROVE YOUR BALANCE

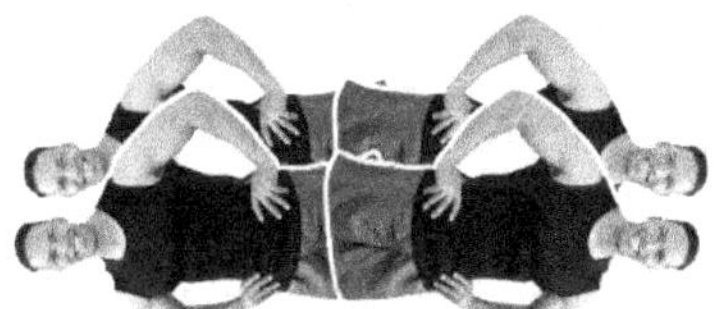

DON'T LET TIME DICTATE YOUR FITNESS, LET FITNESS DEFY TIME

4. ARM CIRCLES

Rotate your arms in small and large circles to improve shoulder mobility.

Starting arm circles is a simple yet effective exercise, especially for older men looking to improve shoulder mobility and flexibility. Arm circles can be performed as part of a warm-up routine or incorporated into a full workout regimen. In this guide, we'll walk you through the steps to properly execute arm circles and highlight their benefits for older individuals.

Step 1: Warm-Up

Warming up your muscles is vital before starting any activity. By doing this, you lower your risk of injury and get your body ready for exercise. To elevate your heart rate and increase blood flow to your muscles, perform light aerobic workouts for 5–10 minutes, such as walking or running.

Step 2: Find a Comfortable Stance

Stand with your feet shoulder-width apart. Maintain good posture by keeping your back straight and your core engaged. This stance provides a stable base for performing arm circles.

Step 3: Proper Hand Placement

At shoulder height, extend your arms out to the sides. Your fingers should be relaxed and your palms should be pointing down. For arm circles, this is the starting position.

Step 4: Small Circles

To begin, initiate small circles with your arms. Imagine drawing circles with your fingertips on a chalkboard. These circles should be about the size of a dinner plate. Perform 10-15 small circles in a forward direction, keeping your movements controlled and deliberate.

Step 5: Reverse Direction

After completing forward circles, reverse the direction. Make 10-15 small circles in a backward direction. Be mindful of your shoulder joints; if you experience any discomfort or pain, reduce the range of motion or stop the exercise.

Step 6: Gradually Increase Circle Size

Once you're comfortable with small circles, gradually increase the size of your circles. Start making larger circles, roughly the size of a hula hoop. Perform 10-15 circles in each direction (forward and backward) with the larger motion.

Step 7: Full Range of Motion

As your shoulder mobility improves, aim to perform arm circles with your arms extended as far as possible. These circles should encompass a full range of motion for your shoulders. Continue with 10-15 circles in both forward and backward directions.

Step 8: Breathing

Remember to breathe steadily throughout the exercise. Inhale and exhale rhythmically to maintain oxygen flow to your muscles. Proper breathing enhances the effectiveness of arm circles and helps you stay relaxed.

Step 9: Cool Down

After completing the desired number of arm circles, lower your arms to your sides and take a moment to cool down. Perform gentle shoulder rolls by rolling your shoulders forward and backward several times. This helps release tension in the shoulder area.

Step 10: Stretch

Finish your routine with shoulder stretches. Gently reach one arm across your chest and hold it with your opposite hand. Hold each stretch for 15-30 seconds on each side to further enhance shoulder flexibility.

Benefits of Arm Circles for Older Men:

- Improved Shoulder Mobility: Arm circles target the shoulder joints, increasing their range of motion and reducing stiffness.

- Enhanced Flexibility: Regularly performing arm circles can help improve overall upper body flexibility.

- Injury Prevention: This exercise helps warm up and strengthen the shoulder muscles, reducing the risk of injuries.

- Better Posture: Increased shoulder mobility contributes to better posture, which is crucial for overall health and comfort.

- Stress Relief: Arm circles can be a relaxing exercise that promotes stress relief through focused, controlled movements.

In conclusion, arm circles are a straightforward yet valuable exercise for older men seeking to enhance their shoulder mobility and flexibility. When done correctly and consistently, they can contribute to improved upper body function and overall well-being. Remember to start with small circles and gradually progress to larger ones to ensure safety and effectiveness. Always listen to your body and consult a healthcare professional if you have any concerns or medical conditions that may affect your ability to perform this exercise.

STRENGTHEN YOUR BODY AND IMPROVE YOUR BALANCE

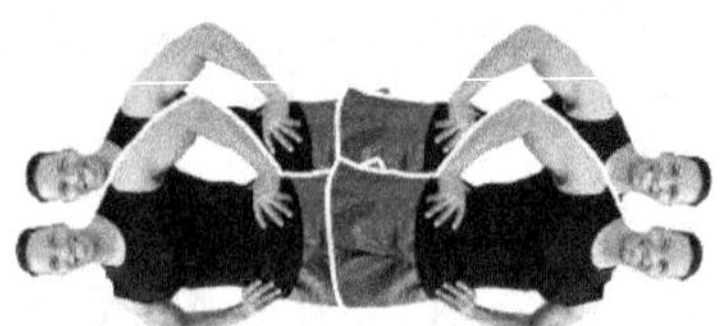

DON'T LET TIME DICTATE YOUR FITNESS, LET FITNESS DEFY TIME

5. TORSO TWISTS

Torso twists are a beneficial exercise for individuals of all ages, but they hold particular advantages for older men looking to enhance core flexibility and maintain overall physical well-being. In this 500-word guide, we'll delve into the step-by-step process of performing torso twists as part of a workout routine tailored to older men.

Step 1: Preparation and Safety

Before initiating any exercise regimen, it's crucial to prioritize safety. For older men, this becomes even more critical. Begin by wearing comfortable workout attire and appropriate footwear. If you have any medical conditions or concerns, consult your healthcare provider before commencing any new exercise program. Ensure you have a clear, spacious area to perform your exercises, free from obstacles or hazards.

Step 2: Proper Stance

To perform torso twists effectively, start by standing with your feet hip-width apart. Your feet should be aligned parallel to each other. Maintaining this stance will provide a stable base to execute the twists and minimize the risk of injury.

Step 3: Hand Placement

Place your hands on your hips or keep them at chest level. This positioning aids in maintaining balance and provides a reference point for the twisting motion.

Step 4: The Twisting Motion

Now, you're ready to initiate the torso twists. Begin by slowly twisting your torso to the left.

Ensure that the movement is controlled and deliberate. The objective is not speed but precision. Gradually return your torso to the center and then twist to the right in the same manner. Perform this twisting motion several times on each side, aiming for at least 10-15 repetitions per set.

Step 5: Breathing Technique

Proper breathing is essential during any exercise. Inhale deeply as you return your torso to the center, and exhale as you twist to each side. This rhythmic breathing pattern helps oxygenate your muscles and maintain focus throughout the exercise.

Step 6: Maintain Good Posture

Maintaining good posture throughout torso twists is crucial for older men. Keep your back straight, shoulders relaxed, and engage your core muscles while twisting. This not only optimizes the effectiveness of the exercise but also reduces the risk of straining your back.

Step 7: Gradual Progression

For older men, it's important to start with a comfortable range of motion and gradually progress. As you become more accustomed to the exercise, you can increase the intensity by twisting a little further or adding light hand weights for resistance.

Step 8: Incorporating Torso Twists into Your Routine

To maximize the benefits of torso twists, incorporate them into a comprehensive workout routine. Older men should focus on a well-rounded fitness program that includes cardiovascular exercises, strength training, and flexibility exercises like torso twists. Aim for at least 2-3 days of strength and flexibility training per week.

Step 9: Listen to Your Body

If you encounter pain, dizziness, or discomfort while completing torso twists, stop immediately and seek medical attention. As with any exercise, it's important to pay attention to your body. You can adjust the range of motion or the number of repetitions to suit your particular fitness level.

Step 10: Cooling Down and Stretching

Spend some time cooling down and stretching your muscles after finishing your torso twists and other exercises. Flexibility is enhanced and muscle soreness is prevented. Include gentle stretches for your back, torso, and core.

In conclusion, torso twists offer older men an effective way to enhance core flexibility and overall fitness. By following these steps, you can perform this exercise safely and effectively as part of a well-rounded workout routine. Always prioritize safety, start slowly, and gradually progress to ensure a sustainable and beneficial fitness journey.

STRENGTHEN YOUR BODY AND IMPROVE YOUR BALANCE

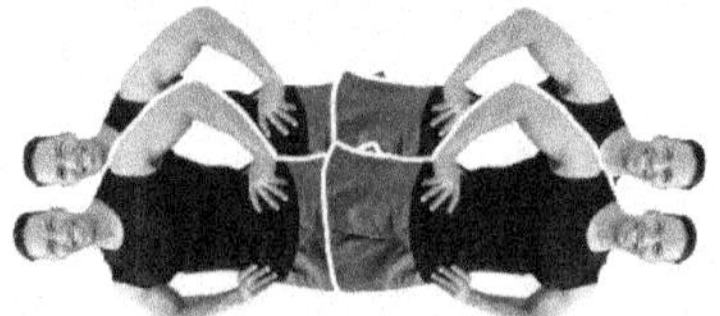

DON'T LET TIME DICTATE YOUR FITNESS, LET FITNESS DEFY TIME

6. SIDE LEG RAISES

As we age, maintaining strength and stability in our hips becomes increasingly important for overall mobility and well-being. One effective exercise for achieving this is the Side Leg Raise. This simple yet impactful exercise targets the hip muscles and can be adapted to various fitness levels. In this guide, we will explore how to perform Side Leg Raises safely and effectively, making it an ideal workout for older men.

Step 1: Preparation

Before beginning any exercise routine, it's crucial to ensure you're adequately prepared. Start by choosing a suitable location where you have enough space to move your legs freely. Wear comfortable clothing and supportive shoes to prevent any slips or discomfort.

Step 2: Equipment

You won't need much equipment for Side Leg Raises, but having a sturdy chair or a wall nearby for balance is highly recommended. This ensures stability and reduces the risk of falls, which is especially important for older individuals.

Step 3: Proper Posture

Stand up straight with your feet hip-width apart. Maintain good posture by keeping your back straight, shoulders relaxed, and chin parallel to the ground. Engaging your core muscles will provide additional support during the exercise.

Step 4: Balance and Support

To perform Side Leg Raises safely, you'll want to hold onto a chair or the wall for balance. Place your hand lightly on the backrest of the chair or the wall at about waist height. This support will help you maintain stability throughout the exercise.

Step 5: Leg Raise Technique

Now, it's time to perform the Side Leg Raises:

- Start with your feet hip-width apart, as mentioned earlier.
- While maintaining a slight bend in your supporting leg, slowly lift your right leg to the side. Keep your toes pointing forward, and make sure your leg is extended but not locked.
- Lift your leg to a comfortable height – it doesn't need to go very high. The goal is to engage your hip muscles.
- Hold the raised position for a second or two, focusing on balance and control. Return

your leg to its initial position by lowering it
slowly.

Step 6: Repetitions and Sets

For beginners or those new to this exercise, start with 10
repetitions for each leg. As you become more comfortable
and confident, gradually increase the number of repetitions
to 15 or 20 per leg. Aim to complete 2-3 sets.

Step 7: Breathing

Don't forget to breathe in time with your movements. As you
raise your leg, inhale; as you lower it, exhale. This deliberate
breathing promotes steadiness and concentration.

Step 8: Safety Tips

Begin with a limited range of motion and progressively
expand it over time. Try not to make jerky motions or
swing your leg.

.

If you experience pain or discomfort, stop immediately and
consult a healthcare professional. Always perform the
exercise in a controlled manner to reduce the risk of injury.

Step 9: Consistency is Key

To experience the full benefits of Side Leg Raises, consistency is essential. Aim to incorporate this exercise into your weekly routine, but be sure to allow your muscles time to rest and recover between sessions.

In conclusion, Side Leg Raises are a valuable addition to the workout routine of older men. They target the hip muscles, promoting strength and stability, which are vital for maintaining mobility as we age. By following these simple steps and safety guidelines, you can perform Side Leg Raises effectively and enjoy the numerous benefits they offer for your overall well-being.

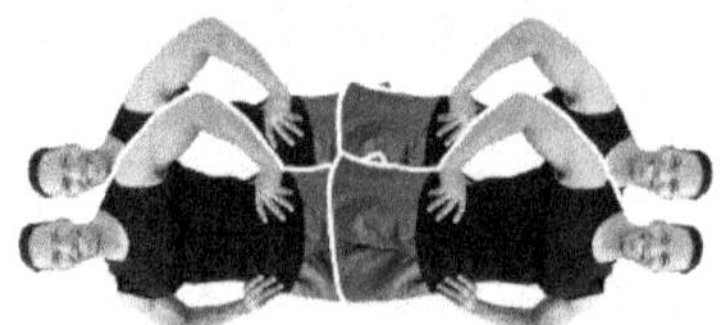

7. LEG SWINGS

To initiate leg swings, a straightforward and effective exercise for enhancing hip and leg mobility, particularly beneficial for older men, follow these steps. Leg swings are a low-impact dynamic stretching exercise that can help improve flexibility, balance, and range of motion in the lower body.

1.Warm-Up: Begin with a brief warm-up to prepare your muscles for the exercise. You can do some light cardio, such as walking or stationary cycling, for 5-10 minutes. This warms up your body and increases blood flow to the muscles.

2. Find a Support: Locate a sturdy support to hold onto while performing leg swings. This could be a wall, a railing, a chair, or any stable object at about waist height. Holding onto support is crucial, especially for older individuals, as it provides balance and prevents falls.

3. Proper Posture: Stand up straight with your feet hip-width apart. Maintain good posture throughout the exercise by keeping your shoulders back and your core engaged. This will help prevent strain on your back and promote better balance.

4.Swing Forward: With one leg, start. For balance, grasp the support with one hand. Take a little step forward with your left leg, keeping it straight but not locked at the knee. Move it forward as far as you are comfortable. The elevated leg's hamstring and hip flexor are the main muscles stretched by this forward movement.

5. Swing Backward: After swinging your leg forward, swing it backward in a controlled manner. As you swing it backward, focus on feeling the stretch in your quadriceps (front thigh) and hip extensors. Keep your movements controlled, and don't force your leg too high.

6. Repeat: Continue swinging your leg forward and backward in a pendulum-like motion for about 10-15 swings on each leg. The goal is to gradually increase the range of motion with each swing, but don't push yourself to the point of discomfort or pain.

7.Switch Legs: After completing the desired number of swings on one leg, switch to the other leg. Remember to maintain your grip on the support for balance.

8.Breathing: Breathing should be done at the same time as leg swinging. Swing your leg forward when exhaling, and backward while inhaling. Your tempo and level of relaxation can both be sustained during the exercise with the aid of this rhythmic breathing.

9. Increase Intensity: As you become more comfortable with leg swings, you can increase the intensity by swinging your leg higher and increasing the number of swings. However, always prioritize safety and control.

10. Cool Down: After you've finished your leg swings on both legs, take a few minutes to cool down with static stretches. Focus on stretching your quadriceps, hamstrings, and hip flexors. Hold each stretch for 15-30 seconds.

11. Frequency: Leg swings can be performed daily or incorporated into your regular workout routine. As you progress, you may find that your balance and range of motion improve, making everyday activities easier and reducing the risk of injury.

12. Listen to Your Body: Pay close attention to how your body feels during leg swings. If you experience pain, dizziness, or discomfort beyond mild stretching sensations, stop the exercise and consult a healthcare professional.

In summary, leg swings are a simple yet effective exercise for improving hip and leg mobility. They can be especially beneficial for older men to maintain flexibility and balance. By following these steps and gradually increasing the intensity over time, you can enjoy the benefits of improved lower body mobility and reduced risk of injury.

STRENGTHEN YOUR BODY AND IMPROVE YOUR BALANCE

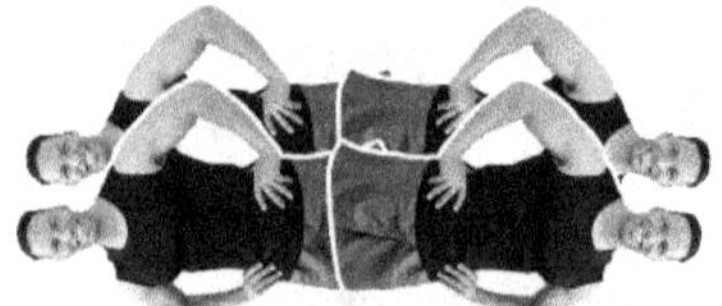

DON'T LET TIME DICTATE YOUR FITNESS, LET FITNESS DEFY TIME

8. KNEE EXTENSIONS

Starting knee extensions while seated is an effective exercise to strengthen the thigh muscles, particularly for older men looking to maintain their leg strength and overall mobility. Knee extensions target the quadriceps, which are crucial for everyday activities like walking, climbing stairs, and maintaining balance. This exercise can be performed with proper form and precautions to ensure safety and effectiveness.

Step 1: Preparation

Before beginning any exercise routine, especially if you're an older individual, it's essential to consult with a healthcare professional or a fitness expert to ensure that knee extensions are suitable for your specific situation. They can provide personalized advice and help you determine the right number of repetitions and sets.

Step 2: Find a Suitable Location

Choose a quiet and comfortable place to perform knee extensions. A sturdy chair without wheels is an excellent option. Ensure that the chair is stable and won't tip over during the exercise.

Step 3: Proper Attire

Wear comfortable clothing and supportive shoes to ensure your safety and comfort while exercising.

Step 4: Warm-Up

Always warm up your muscles for a few minutes before working out. A few minutes of marching in place, light leg swings, and ankle circles can assist to improve blood flow to the muscles and lower the chance of injury.

Step 5: Seating Position

Your feet should be hip-width apart while you sit on the chair with your back straight. Your thighs should be parallel to the ground and your knees should be bent 90 degrees.

Step 6: Starting the Knee Extensions

- Place your hands on the sides of the chair or grasp the armrests for stability.
- Begin by extending one leg straight in front of you, raising your foot a few inches off the ground. Your heel should be in line with your knee.
- Hold the extended position for a moment, focusing on contracting your quadriceps muscles.
- Slowly lower your foot back to the starting position, ensuring controlled and deliberate movement. Avoid any jerky or rapid motions.

- Repeat the same process with your other leg.

Step 7: Breathing

Exhale as you extend your leg and inhale as you return to the starting position. Maintaining proper breathing throughout the exercise is important for providing your muscles with oxygen and reducing the risk of fatigue.

Step 8: Repetitions and Sets

Starting with 10 to 15 repetitions each leg is a manageable quantity to start with. As you become more accustomed to the workout, gradually up the repetitions. In each workout, aim for two to three sets.

Step 9: Monitoring Progress

Keep a workout journal to track your progress. Note the number of repetitions, sets, and any discomfort or pain you may experience. This journal can help you adjust your routine over time.

Step 10: Cool Down

After completing your knee extensions, take a few minutes to cool down. Gentle stretches for your quadriceps and hamstrings can be beneficial in preventing muscle soreness.

Step 11: Safety Considerations

- When extending your knees, stop immediately if you feel any pain, and seek medical advice.

- To prevent strain or damage, keep perfect form throughout the entire workout.
- When stretching your legs, avoid locking your knees. To protect the joint, keep your knees slightly bent.

- Progress gradually. Don't push yourself too hard too soon.

In conclusion, seated knee extensions are a valuable exercise for older men to strengthen their thigh muscles and improve overall leg strength. By following these steps with care and patience, you can incorporate knee extensions into your fitness routine safely and effectively, promoting better mobility and quality of life as you age.

9. CALF RAISES

Calf raises are a simple yet effective exercise that can help older men improve lower leg strength and stability. To perform calf raises safely and effectively, follow these steps:

Warm-Up: Warming up your muscles is crucial before beginning any training activity. Spend 5–10 minutes doing easy cardio workouts like stationary cycling or walking. Your muscles will receive more blood flow, which will better prepare them for exercise.

Foot Position: Begin by standing with your feet hip-width apart. Ensure that your weight is evenly distributed between both feet to maintain balance and stability.

Body Posture: Maintain a straight spine throughout the workout. Keep your core tight, your shoulders back, and your chest high. By doing this, you can avoid lower back stress.

Use Support: If you have trouble with balance, it's a good idea to use a sturdy support like a wall, chair, or countertop to hold onto lightly. This can help you maintain your balance during the exercise.

Execution: Now, you're ready to start the calf raises:

a) Lift Your Heels: To start, gradually raise your heels off the floor. Keep your attention on pressing through the balls of your feet.

b) Rise Onto Your Toes: Up until you are standing on your tiptoes, keep elevating your heels.

c) Your calf muscles need to begin to contract at this moment.

d) Hold and Squeeze: Hold the position for a moment after you've lifted as high as you can without feeling uncomfortable. To increase the contraction, squeeze your calves.

e) Lower Your Heels: Slowly lower your heels back down to the starting position. Ensure you do this in a controlled manner; don't let your heels drop quickly.

f) Repetitions and Sets: Aim for 2-3 sets of 10-15 repetitions to begin with. The number of sets or repetitions can be gradually increased as you get more accustomed to the activity.

h) Breathing: Pay attention to your breathing. Inhale as you lift your heels, and exhale as you lower them. This rhythmic breathing can help you maintain control and prevent dizziness.

i) Progression: As your calf muscles strengthen, you can make the exercise more challenging. You can do this by holding onto weights (dumbbells or a backpack filled with books) or performing single-leg calf raises for added difficulty.

j) Stretch: After completing your calf raises, it's essential to stretch your calf muscles. This can be done by placing your hands on a wall and gently leaning forward, keeping your heel on the ground, and feeling the stretch in your calf. Hold this stretch for 15-30 seconds on each leg.

k) Cool Down: Finish your calf raise workout with a few minutes of light stretching or walking to gradually bring your heart rate down.

Remember, it's crucial to listen to your body. If you experience pain or discomfort during calf raises, stop immediately and consult a healthcare professional or fitness expert. Always start with a manageable level of intensity and gradually increase it as your strength improves. Calf raises, when performed correctly, can be a valuable addition to an older man's workout routine, helping to strengthen the lower legs and improve balance

STRENGTHEN YOUR BODY AND IMPROVE YOUR BALANCE

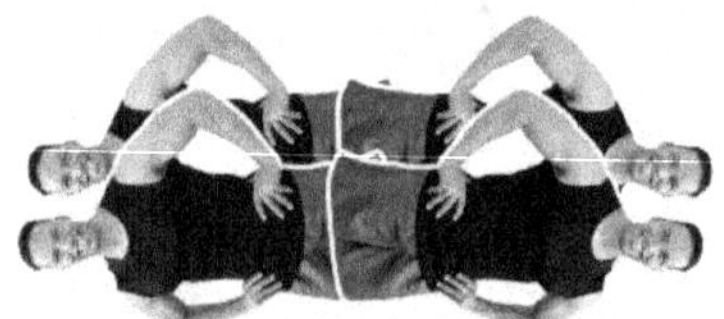

DON'T LET TIME DICTATE YOUR FITNESS, LET FITNESS DEFY TIME

10.WALL PUSH-UPS

Wall push-ups are a simple yet effective exercise that can help older men strengthen their chest and arms while minimizing the risk of injury. This low-impact workout is especially suitable for those who may have joint issues or limited mobility. In this guide, we will outline how to start wall push-ups as part of a fitness routine tailored to the needs of older men.

1. Preparation and Safety:

Before beginning any exercise routine, it's essential to prioritize safety. Consult with a healthcare professional, especially if you have any pre-existing medical conditions or concerns about your ability to perform physical activities. Once you have the green light, choose a
location with a sturdy wall that is clear of obstacles and provides enough space for you to extend your arms fully.

2. Warm-Up

Always start with a warm-up to prepare your muscles for exercise. A light five to ten-minute cardio activity, like brisk walking or stationary cycling, can increase blood flow to your muscles and reduce the risk of strains or injuries.

3. Proper Body Alignment:

Standing with your feet shoulder-width apart, face the wall. Engage your core muscles while maintaining a straight back. To avoid putting undue strain on your back, keep a proper posture throughout the workout.

4. Hand Placement

Place your hands on the wall at shoulder height, slightly wider than shoulder-width apart. Your palms should be flat against the wall, and your fingers should be pointing upward.

5. The Push-Up Motion

Slowly bend your elbows while keeping your body in a straight line. Lower your chest towards the wall until your nose almost touches it. Ensure that your elbows point outwards and away from your body as you descend.

6. Controlled Movement

Controlled push-ups should be done while concentrating on the contraction of your arm and chest muscles. As you push up against the wall to go back to where you started, exhale. Although your arms should be fully extended, keep your elbows loose.

7. Repetitions and Sets

Start with a manageable number of repetitions, such as 10 to 15, for one set. As your strength and confidence improve, gradually increase the number of repetitions and sets. Aim to work up to three sets of 15 to 20 repetitions.

8. Breathing

Throughout the workout, breathe in a steady, controlled way. Exhale as you push away from the wall while inhaling as you lower your chest toward it.

9. Rest and Recovery

Allow your muscles time to recover between sets. Take a brief break, about 30 seconds to a minute, before starting the next set. This rest period helps prevent overexertion and maintains proper form.

10. Progression

As you become more comfortable with wall push-ups, you can increase the challenge by stepping farther away from the wall, which increases the angle of your body. A greater angle requires more strength to push your body weight. Alternatively, you can explore other push-up variations, such as incline or decline push-ups, to continue progressing.

11. Cool Down

Perform a cool-down regimen that includes chest, arm, and shoulder stretches after finishing your sets. This lessens muscular pain and increases flexibility.

12. Consistency

Consistency is key to reaping the benefits of wall push-ups. Aim to incorporate this exercise into your fitness routine at least two to three times a week. As your strength improves, you may want to diversify your workout with additional exercises to target different muscle groups.

In summary, wall push-ups are a safe and effective way for older men to strengthen their chest and arms. By following these steps and gradually increasing the intensity, you can build muscle strength and improve your overall fitness while minimizing the risk of injury. Remember to consult with a healthcare professional before starting any new exercise program, especially if you have underlying health concerns.

11. CHAIR SQUATS

Chair squats are a beneficial exercise, especially for older men looking to strengthen their legs and glutes while improving balance and mobility. In this guide, we'll provide a step-by-step explanation of how to start chair squats:

Chair squats are a seated-to-standing exercise that can be done without using your hands for support. They are ideal for individuals who may have limited mobility or strength but still want to work on lower body strength.

Step 1: Preparation

- Choose a Sturdy Chair: Begin by selecting a sturdy, stable chair with a solid backrest. Avoid chairs with wheels or those that are too soft, as they may not provide the necessary support.

- Proper Foot Position: Sit towards the front of the chair, ensuring your feet are flat on the ground and hip-width apart. Your knees should be aligned with your ankles, forming a 90-degree angle.

- Engage Your Core: Before you start, engage your core muscles by pulling your belly button toward your spine.

This will help you maintain stability throughout the exercise.

Step 2: Perform the Chair Squat

- Initiate the Movement: To begin the squat, shift your weight forward slightly. Focus on pushing through your heels as you slowly stand up without using your hands for support. Keep your chest lifted and your back straight throughout the movement.

- Controlled Descent: As you stand, exhale and maintain control over your movement. Imagine sitting back down into the chair.

- Proper Form: Pay close attention to your form. Your knees should remain aligned with your ankles, and your back should not round or arch excessively. Keep your chest up, and avoid leaning forward.

- Depth: Aim to lower yourself until your hips are just above the chair. Don't plop down; instead, lower yourself with control.

- Repetition: Start with a manageable number of repetitions, perhaps 8-10, and gradually increase as you become more comfortable with the exercise.

Step 3: Safety and Tips

- Safety First: If you experience pain or discomfort while performing chair squats, stop immediately. Consult with a healthcare professional if you have any concerns about your ability to perform this exercise safely.

- Use a Spotter: If you're unsure about your balance or strength, it's a good idea to have someone nearby to assist you, especially when you're first starting.

- Warm-Up: Always begin your exercise routine with a proper warm-up to prepare your muscles for the activity. Gentle leg stretches and ankle circles can be helpful.

- Gradual Progression: Aim to gradually increase your squats' repetitions and, if you can, their depth. You can keep your muscles challenged in this way.

- Regular Practice: Consistency is key. Aim to incorporate chair squats into your workout routine on a regular basis to see improvements in leg and glute strength.

In summary, chair squats are an effective exercise for older men looking to strengthen their legs and glutes while maintaining balance and mobility. By following these steps and incorporating proper form and safety precautions, you can safely begin chair squats as part of your workout routine. Remember to start slowly, gradually increase intensity, and consult a healthcare professional if you have any concerns about your fitness level or any underlying medical conditions.

STRENGTHEN YOUR BODY AND IMPROVE YOUR BALANCE

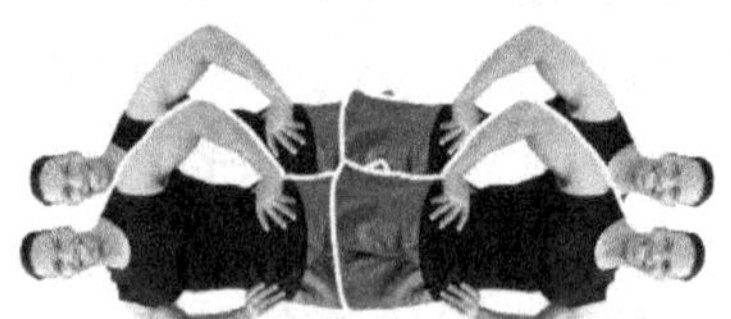

DON'T LET TIME DICTATE YOUR FITNESS, LET FITNESS DEFY TIME

12. STEP-UPS

As we age, maintaining lower body strength and balance becomes increasingly important for overall health and independence. One effective exercise to achieve these goals is the step-up. This comprehensive guide will walk older men through the process of starting step-ups using a stable step or low bench. Step-ups are a versatile and accessible exercise that can be adapted to various fitness levels and needs.

1. Safety First

Before diving into any exercise routine, safety should be a top priority, especially for older individuals. Consult with a healthcare professional or a certified trainer to ensure that step-ups are safe and appropriate for your specific circumstances. They can provide guidance tailored to your unique needs and limitations.

2. Equipment Preparation

To begin step-ups, you'll need a stable step or a low bench. Choose a step that is sturdy, non-slip, and about knee-height or slightly lower. Make sure it's positioned on a flat surface to prevent any wobbling or instability during the exercise.

3. Warm-Up

To prepare your muscles and joints, a comprehensive warm-up is crucial. To improve blood flow and loosen up your body, spend 5 to 10 minutes performing modest aerobic workouts like brisk walking or stationary cycling..

4. Proper Footwear

Wear comfortable, supportive athletic shoes with good traction to reduce the risk of slipping or losing balance while performing step-ups.

5. Correct Form

In order to minimize injuries and maximize the benefits of the exercise, it is essential to maintain appropriate form. Here is a step-by-step explanation of the right format:

- Stand in front of the step with your feet hip-width apart.
- Engage your core muscles for stability.
- Place one foot flat on the step, ensuring that your entire foot is on the surface.
- Push through your heel and engage your glutes and quadriceps as you step up onto the platform.
- Carefully step back down with the opposite foot, returning to the starting position.
- Repeat the process for the desired number of repetitions on each leg.

6. Breathing

Inhale as you step up and exhale as you step back down. Proper breathing helps maintain oxygen flow to your muscles and supports stability.

7. Start Slow

If you're new to step-ups or have been inactive for a while, begin with a low step and a small number of repetitions. Gradually increase the step height and the number of reps as your strength and balance improve.

8. Progression

To continue benefiting from step-ups, increase the challenge over time. This can be achieved by adding weights, increasing step height, or incorporating variations like lateral step-ups or step-ups with knee raises.

9. Cool Down

After completing your step-up session, cool down by stretching your lower body muscles. Focus on the calves, quadriceps, hamstrings, and hip flexors. Hold each stretch for 15-30 seconds.

10. Listen to Your Body

Pay close attention to how your body responds to step-ups. If you experience pain, dizziness, or discomfort beyond normal muscle fatigue, stop immediately and seek advice from a healthcare professional.

11. Consistency is Key

Consistency is crucial for step-ups to be successful. Aim for at least two to three workouts per week, gradually escalating the length and difficulty of your sessions as you advance.

12. Monitor Progress

To keep track of your improvement, keep an exercise journal. Take note of the repetitions performed, the height of the steps, and any additional weights used. You can use this to set goals and track your progress.

In summary, step-ups are an excellent exercise for older men looking to enhance lower body strength and balance. By following these guidelines and emphasizing safety, proper form, and gradual progression, you can incorporate step-ups into your fitness routine and enjoy the many benefits they offer for overall health and well-being. Remember, it's never too late to start working on your physical fitness, and step-ups are a simple yet effective way to do just that.

13. PLANKS

Planks are an excellent exercise for building core strength and stability, making them a valuable addition to a workout routine, especially for older men. To start incorporating planks into your fitness regimen, follow these steps:

1. Preparation: Before you begin any exercise routine, it's crucial to consult with a healthcare professional, especially if you have any pre-existing medical conditions or concerns. Once you get the green light to start, you can proceed with confidence.

2. Find a Suitable Surface: Choose a flat, comfortable surface for performing planks. A yoga mat or a carpeted area can provide cushioning for your elbows and help prevent discomfort.

3. Warm-Up: Always warm up your body before attempting any exercise. Spend 5-10 minutes doing light aerobic activities like walking or gentle stretching to increase blood flow to your muscles.

5. Correct Form: Proper form is essential for the effectiveness of planks and to avoid injury. To begin, get into a push-up position, but instead of placing your hands on the ground, rest your weight on your forearms. Keep your elbows directly beneath your shoulders and your forearms parallel to each other.

6. Alignment: Make sure your body is aligned in a straight line from head to heels. Pulling your navel toward your spine will help you to activate your core muscles. This protects your lower back while simultaneously strengthening your core.

7. Leg Position: Your toes should be tucked under, and your feet should be hip-width apart. Distribute your weight evenly between your forearms and toes.

8. Breathing: Remember to breathe deeply. Exhale via your mouth after taking a big breath through your nose. During the activity, keep breathing steadily.

9. Duration: Start with a reasonable timeframe. A decent place to start for novices is holding a plank for 20–30 seconds. Increase the time gradually as you advance. Attempt to go as long as a minute.

10. Avoid Overarching or Sagging: Maintain a straight line from head to heels throughout the plank. Avoid raising your hips too high or letting them sink toward the ground.

11. Engage Muscles: Concentrate on engaging your core muscles throughout the exercise. You should feel tension in your abdominals, not in your lower back or shoulders.

12. Rest and Repeat: After holding the plank for your chosen duration, gently lower yourself to the ground. Rest for a minute or so and then repeat the exercise for 2-3 sets.

13. Progression: As your strength improves, you can make planks more challenging by trying variations. Side planks, plank leg lifts, or plank with shoulder taps are all great options.

14. Consistency: Incorporate planks into your workout routine 2-3 times a week. Consistency is key to seeing improvements in core strength and stability.

15. Listen to Your Body: Pay attention to how your body responds. If you experience pain or discomfort beyond

normal muscle fatigue, stop immediately and consult a healthcare professional.

16. Cool Down: Spend a few minutes stretching your core and other significant muscle areas after your planking practice. Flexibility is increased, and muscle pain is lessened.

In summary, starting planks for core strength and stability involves proper preparation, form, and gradual progression. Consistency and patience are essential, and always prioritize safety and listening to your body. Planks can be an effective and accessible exercise for older men looking to enhance their overall fitness and functional strength.

STRENGTHEN YOUR BODY AND IMPROVE YOUR BALANCE

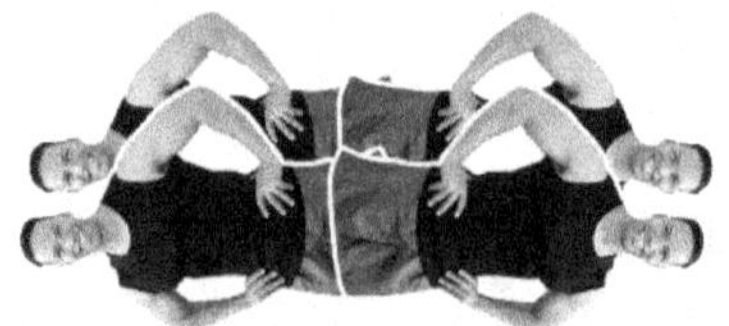

DON'T LET TIME DICTATE YOUR FITNESS, LET FITNESS DEFY TIME

14. SEATED LEG LIFTS

Maintaining a healthy, active lifestyle becomes more crucial as we get older. Exercise is essential in this process because it maintains muscle mass, improves balance, and improves general wellbeing. For older men, seated leg lifts are a great addition to a fitness regimen because they target the lower abdomen muscles while providing a low-impact, secure exercise. This article will cover how to begin sitting leg lifts, highlighting their significance and outlining a step-by-step procedure.

Importance of Seated Leg Lifts for Older Men

Before delving into the exercise itself, it's crucial to understand why seated leg lifts are valuable for older men. These lifts focus on the lower abdominal muscles, a region often weakened with age. By strengthening these muscles, individuals can experience numerous benefits:

1.Improved Core Stability: A strong core is essential for maintaining balance and preventing falls, which can be particularly dangerous for older adults.

2.Enhanced Mobility: Strong lower abdominal muscles assist in daily activities like standing up from a chair or climbing stairs.

3.Back Pain Prevention: Strengthening the core can alleviate lower back pain, a common issue among older individuals.

4.Better Posture: A stable core promotes better posture, reducing the risk of hunching or stooping.

Now, let's outline a step-by-step guide on how to start seated leg lifts.

Step 1: Find a Sturdy Chair

Begin by selecting a sturdy, armless chair with a flat seat. This chair will provide the support you need while allowing your legs to move freely.

Step 2: Sit Upright

Your feet should be flat on the floor and hip-width apart as you sit in the chair, toward the front edge. Keep your shoulders relaxed and your back straight in an upright position.

Step 3: Hand Placement

Place your hands on the sides of the chair seat to stabilize yourself. This will also help you maintain balance throughout the exercise.

Step 4: Leg Lifts

- Now, you're ready to perform the leg lifts:
- Start with your right leg. Slowly lift it straight out in front of you, keeping your foot flexed. Aim to raise it to hip level or as high as comfortably possible.
- Hold your leg in this raised position for a few seconds, engaging your lower abdominal muscles.
- Gently lower your right leg back down to the floor.
- Repeat this process with your left leg.

Step 5: Repetitions and Sets

Begin with a manageable number of repetitions, such as 5-10 lifts per leg. As you become more comfortable with the exercise, gradually increase the repetitions and sets.

Step 6: Breathing

Keep your breathing even while you perform the workout. As you raise your leg, inhale; as you lower it, exhale.

Step 7: Safety First

Always put safety first. If you feel any pain or discomfort while exercising, stop right away. It's critical to pay attention to your body's signals and avoid overexerting yourself.

Conclusion

Seated leg lifts are a valuable addition to the workout routine of older men. By targeting the lower abdominal muscles, they contribute to core stability, mobility, posture, and back pain prevention. This simple exercise can be performed at home with a sturdy chair, making it accessible to many. As with any exercise program, it's advisable to consult a healthcare professional before starting, especially if you have underlying health conditions. With dedication and consistency, seated leg lifts can help older men enjoy a more active and fulfilling life.

STRENGTHEN YOUR BODY AND IMPROVE YOUR BALANCE

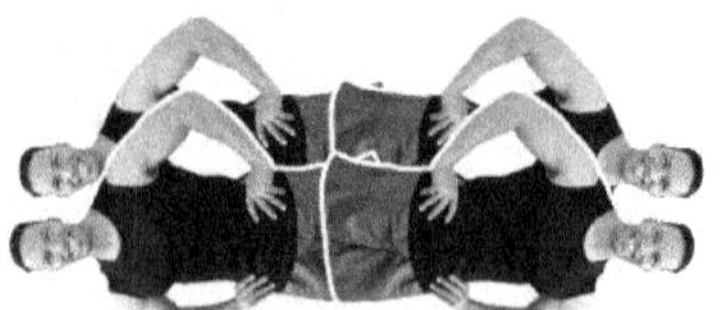

DON'T LET TIME DICTATE YOUR FITNESS, LET FITNESS DEFY TIME

15. COOL DOWN AND STRETCHING

Cooling down and stretching are crucial components of any workout, especially for older men. They help improve flexibility, reduce muscle tension, and prevent injury. In this guide, we'll explain how to properly cool down and stretch after a workout, tailored to the needs of older men.

Why Cool Down and Stretch?

Cooling down and stretching serve several important purposes, especially for older individuals:

1. Reducing Muscle Stiffness: As we age, our muscles tend to stiffen up. Stretching post-workout helps combat this stiffness.

2. Improving Flexibility: Flexibility decreases with age, but regular stretching can help maintain and even improve it.

3. Preventing Injury: Cooling down gradually lowers your heart rate and stretching helps prevent muscle strains and joint injuries.

Cool Down (5-10 minutes):

1. **Slow Your Pace:** After completing the main part of your workout, gradually reduce your intensity. If you've been running, start walking; if lifting weights, use lighter weights.

2. **Hydration:** Take small sips of water to rehydrate. Dehydration can lead to muscle cramps and injuries.

3. **Deep Breathing**: Focus on deep, controlled breaths to bring your heart rate down. Inhale through your nose for a count of four, hold for four, and exhale for four.

4. **Keep Moving**: Perform low-intensity exercises like brisk walking or gentle cycling for 5-10 minutes. This helps prevent blood pooling in your legs.

Stretching (10-15 minutes)

1.Start with Dynamic Stretches: Dynamic stretches, which involve controlled motions, are a good place to start. Leg swings, arm circles, and hip rotations are a few examples. Your muscles will be ready for static stretching after these.

2. Static Stretching: For 15 to 30 seconds, hold each stretch. Prioritize the main muscular groups, including:

- Quadriceps: Stand and hold your ankle behind you, pulling gently toward your buttocks.

- Hamstrings: Sit on the floor, one leg extended, and reach for your toes.

- Chest: Clasp your hands behind your back and gently pull your arms upward.

- Shoulders: Cross one arm across your chest and gently pull it with the opposite hand.

- Calves: Lean against a wall with one foot forward, keeping the back leg straight.

3. Avoid Bouncing: Never bounce while stretching. This can lead to muscle strains.

4. Stretch the Core: Focus on the core by doing gentle torso twists and side stretches. A strong core is essential for balance and stability, which are crucial for older individuals.

5. Breathe and Relax: Continue your deep, controlled breathing while you stretch. Don't force the stretch; simply relax into it.

6. Balance and Flexibility: Include balance exercises like yoga poses. These can improve flexibility and stability, which are essential for preventing falls.

7.Target Problem Areas: Pay extra attention to areas where you feel tightness or discomfort. Be cautious and gentle, especially if you have any preexisting injuries.

Listen to Your Body:

Keep in mind that every person has a unique body, so what works for one person could not work for someone else. If you feel any pain when stretching, stop right away. Stretching shouldn't hurt, just be a little uncomfortable.

.

STRENGTHEN YOUR BODY AND IMPROVE YOUR BALANCE

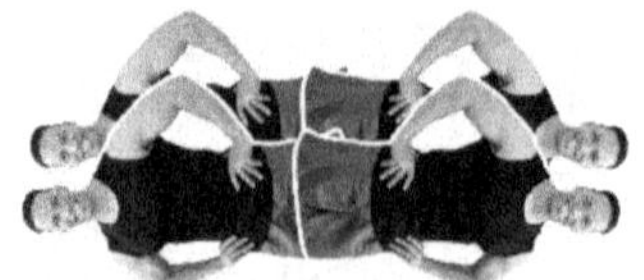

DON'T LET TIME DICTATE YOUR FITNESS, LET FITNESS DEFY TIME

CONCLUSION

In summary, a morning fitness regimen designed specifically for older men is more than simply a routine; it's a means to improve overall wellbeing and have a satisfying life in your golden years. This all-encompassing strategy addresses the particular physical and mental requirements of senior citizens by incorporating flexibility exercises, weight training, and cardiovascular activities.

Older men can strengthen their cardiovascular system, increase endurance, and efficiently manage their weight by regularly engaging in cardiovascular workouts like brisk walking or cycling. In addition, including strength training exercises, such as bodyweight exercises or small weights, helps maintain valuable muscle mass and bone density, counteracting the loss of both due to aging.

Aside from maintaining joint mobility, including flexibility activities like yoga or stretching also encourages relaxation and stress reduction. This trifecta of physical activity benefits not just mental but also physical health, promoting a happy view on life.

We provide the following special inspiration to our readers: Accept this early workout as part of your regular routine.

Recognize that the advantages go far beyond the physical; they also include regaining vigor, maintaining an active lifestyle, and appreciating each day to the fullest. You have the chance to shatter preconceived notions about aging by continuing to be nimble, resilient, and mentally sharp.

Include this practice in your life as a celebration of your wellbeing rather than as a requirement. Let it serve as a reminder of your resolve to live a life well-lived, one in which every daybreak holds up the promise of renewed vigor and limitless possibilities. Never forget that starting is never too late and that the benefits are endless. So get up and shine because you have the chance each morning to change the course of your life through the power of regular exercise.

STRENGTHEN YOUR BODY AND IMPROVE YOUR BALANCE

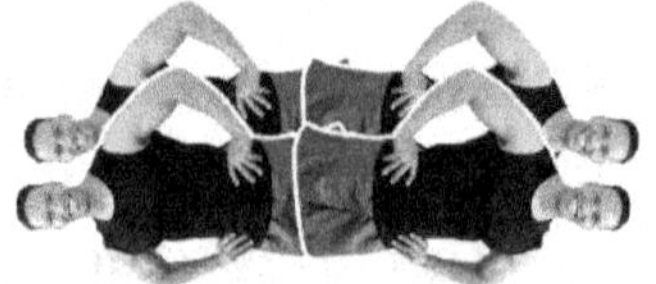

DON'T LET TIME DICTATE YOUR FITNESS, LET FITNESS DEFY TIME

We appreciate you choosing to follow our daily morning fitness plan for older men as you set out on your path to a healthier, happier you. Your dedication to taking care of yourself is greatly appreciated.

Keep in mind that even the smallest step you take toward living a healthier lifestyle counts as progress. Making the choice to put your health first is a gift to both you and your loved ones. You're making an investment in a more robust future by setting aside your mornings for these exercises.

We hope that this guide has motivated you to value self-care, perseverance, and routine. Remember that you're not alone in your endeavor; there are others out there who share your desire to improve on each passing day.

Your commitment to protecting your health, which is a priceless possession, is remarkable. So, be aware that you're making progress toward a more contented and active existence every morning as you lace up your sneakers, unfold your yoga mat, or grab those weights. We appreciate your decision to put your health and wellbeing first. Keep up the good work, and may each day bring you a little bit closer to the full, active, and happy life you so richly deserve. Here's to many more energizing and vibrant sunrises!

WORKOUT JOURNAL

DATE_______________________

MY WORKOUT

MY GOAL

MY NOTE

WORKOUT JOURNAL

DATE________________

MY WORKOUT

MY GOAL

MY NOTE

DATE________________

MY WORKOUT

MY GOAL

MY NOTE

WORKOUT JOURNAL

DATE_______________________

MY WORKOUT

MY GOAL

MY NOTE

WORKOUT JOURNAL

DATE______________________

MY WORKOUT

MY GOAL

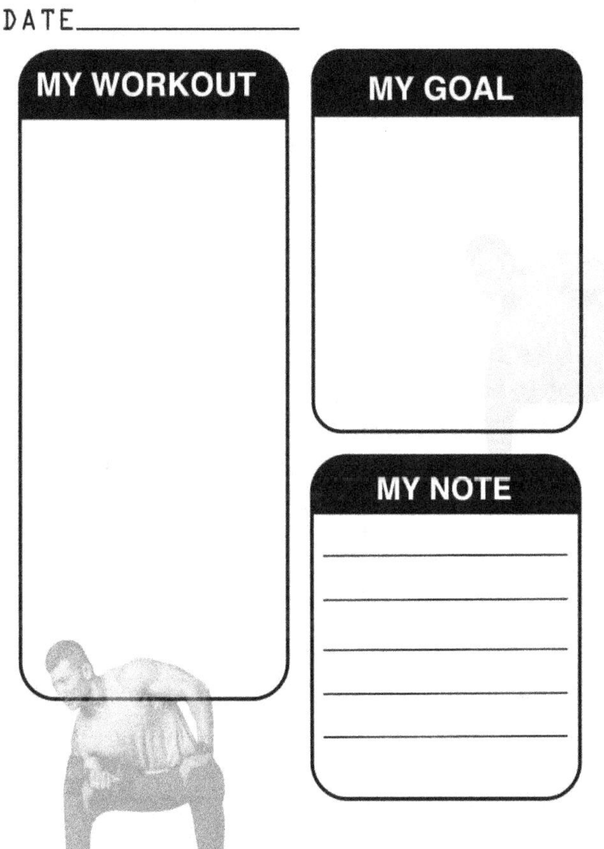

MY NOTE

DATE_______________________

MY WORKOUT

MY GOAL

MY NOTE

WORKOUT JOURNAL

DATE__________________

MY WORKOUT

MY GOAL

MY NOTE

WORKOUT JOURNAL

DATE________________

MY WORKOUT

MY GOAL

MY NOTE

WORKOUT JOURNAL

DATE________________

MY WORKOUT

MY GOAL

MY NOTE

WORKOUT JOURNAL

DATE_________________

MY WORKOUT

MY GOAL

MY NOTE

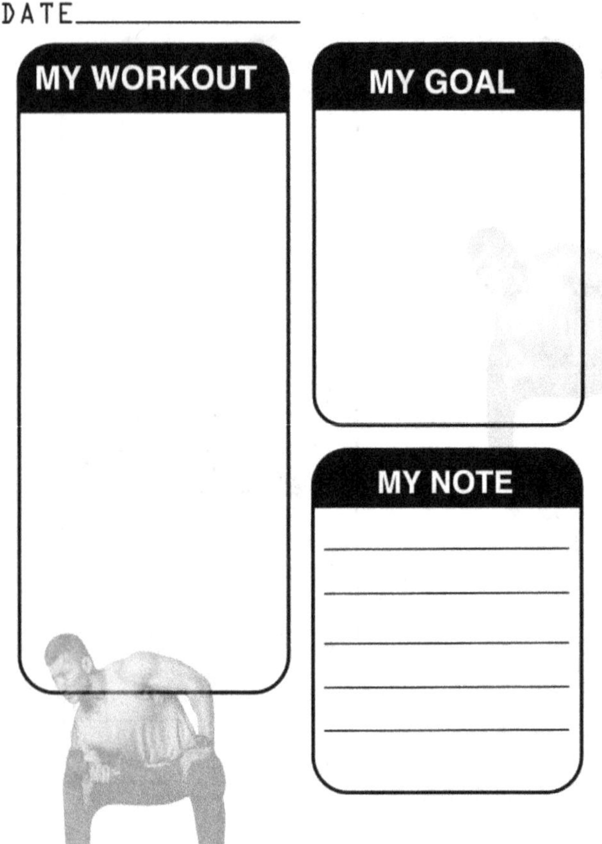

WORKOUT JOURNAL

DATE___________________

MY WORKOUT

MY GOAL

MY NOTE

WORKOUT JOURNAL

DATE_______________________

MY WORKOUT

MY GOAL

MY NOTE